MILLICENT NYANGON

Bounce Back

My Battle With Systemic Lupus

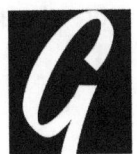

First published by GREAT Books 2020

Copyright © 2020 by Millicent Nyangon

All rights reserved. No part of this publication may be reproduced, stored or transmitted in any form or by any means, electronic, mechanical, photocopying, recording, scanning, or otherwise without written permission from the publisher. It is illegal to copy this book, post it to a website, or distribute it by any other means without permission.

Millicent Nyangon asserts the moral right to be identified as the author of this work.

All Scripture quotations, unless otherwise indicated, are taken from the Holy Bible, New International Version®, NIV®. Copyright ©1973, 1978, 1984, 2011 by Biblica, Inc.™ Used by permission of Zondervan. All rights reserved worldwide. www.zondervan.comThe "NIV" and "New International Version" are trademarks registered in the United States Patent and Trademark Office by Biblica, Inc.™

First edition

This book was professionally typeset on Reedsy. Find out more at reedsy.com

Contents

Introduction	iv
The Ability to Bounce Back	vi
1 The Symptoms and the Testing of My Faith	1
2 The Visit To The Doctor	3
3 The Wait	9
4 The Process of Diagnosis	12
5 The Process of Recovery	14
6 Lessons Learned	21
Unwavering Faith	23
Never Take Life for Granted	24

Introduction

By Simon Nyangon

You must have heard " tough times never seem to end" especially when a family member becomes sick with a life-threatening disease or a disease that is classified as not having a cure and can only be managed. In 2015, we lost my father in law when my wife was in the middle of finalizing a double major. She had to travel to Kenya to attend her Daddy's burial in the midst of her final exams As a strong woman, she never showed any signs of fatigue until three months after her graduation. What looked like fatigue, escalated to what looked like a skin allergy, to hair falling out, and was later diagnosed as lupus.

None of us saw any hope of recovery, and it became worse as time went by. We witnessed what we had never seen before in her life, loss of muscles that translated to hanging pockets of skin, loss of regular sleep that couldn't be controlled, and her skin losing oil and becoming scaly. The journey to recovery was long and difficult and as a husband and a close friend I had to do what it took to help my wife in her fight. It was one of the toughest times our family has had to endure and I kept on saying "this too shall pass" to encourage myself

However, despite the odds against her, my wife soon developed confidence and never viewed anything as a loss but always saw a light at the end of the tunnel. The long days that turned out to be three years seemed to have shortened with time and as a family, this sense of optimism became our new normal. Thanks to our close friends who regularly came to encourage us and pray with us. Their encouragement and presence in our home gave my wife the opportunity to crack her favorite jokes and tell stories and that became therapeutic for her and helped to turn the tides of lupus.

Whenever we visited the hospital, she always left the doctors and nurses encouraged even though the tests were pointing south. Her belief of a total recovery was unquestionable and the doctors and nurses had no doubt she would recover. Some of the nurses and doctors and wished that she would be given a chance to encourage some of their other patients. When the recovery started, it was speedy and dramatic and it didn't take long before her body began to show improvement. The bloodwork and tests also showed improvement and my wife was back.

In conclusion, I do not wish this experience on anyone and to date, I still find it difficult to reflect on those days or even look at pictures we took as documentation of my wife's illness. My prayer is that her story will fill your hearts with hope and conviction that with God, all things are possible.

The Ability to Bounce Back

My Journey

"Happy New Year" is what we all tell each other any time a New Year begins, with the hope that the new year will be better than the previous year and bring with it new hope and greater experiences new year resolutions are made, vision boards are put up, and we get to work to achieve them. No one prepares for failure, sickness, or any sort of calamity.

Therefore when 2016 rolled in, naturally I was looking forward to a great year. 2015 had ended on a bittersweet note. Bitter because my Dad passed away in November, and sweet because I graduated with a double major in Organizational Communication and Political Science in December. Unfortunately, three months into the year, the unexpected happened.

Here's my story.

1

The Symptoms and the Testing of My Faith

In the spring of 2016, I noticed a rash on the tip of my nose. I did not worry about it at first, but after a few days, I noticed that it was spreading and that there was something different with the size of my nose. So, I decided to take a selfie and compare it to my old pictures. It was evident that my nose had significantly increased in size. This was the strangest thing I had ever seen. How does the nose just grow?

I called my long time friend Liz and told her that it looked like my nose was growing.

"You're not serious," she laughed.

To prove to her that I was not joking, I hung up and sent her the picture. She immediately called me back. This time she was no longer laughing.

"Millicent, you need to call your Doctor immediately," she suggested.

I assured her that I would.

When my husband came back from work, I showed him the picture I had taken during the day and compared it to a previous picture. Seeing the two pictures side by side, he also agreed that something was going on and suggested that I make an appointment to see my Primary Clinical Physician (PCP).

April 2016

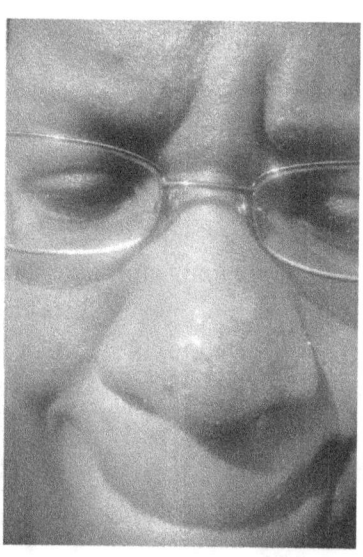

2

The Visit To The Doctor

The next morning, I called the doctor and made an appointment for both my husband because we were due for our annual check-up. I figured we might as well kill two birds with one stone. After seeing the rashes, the doctor concluded that it might be allergies since it was Spring, and advised that I buy Claritin from the pharmacy. The interesting thing is, since 2001 the year my family and I came to the USA, until that day, I had never taken Claritin or had any allergies. Therefore, I found it strange that all of a sudden I had developed allergies.

After the doctor concluded that I had a simple case of allergy, she proceeded to conduct our annual physical examinations which included blood work. The doctor informed us that we would get a call when she received the results of the blood work so that we could discuss them.

A few days passed, and it looked like the longer we waited the bigger my nose grew, and the rashes spread from my nose to both my eyebrows. At this point, my eyebrows were falling out. This no longer looked like an allergy. It looked terrible, and it was itching. The fact that my nose was growing was alarming.

"How big will it grow?"

"Why is it growing?"

These were the questions that were running through my mind. The doctor finally called after a week and told us that our blood work was normal.

"How can it be normal?" I exclaimed.

I explained to her that not only was my nose still growing but that the rashes had spread to both my eyebrows and in fact, my eyebrows had fallen out.

"What in the world was happening to me?" I asked the doctor.

"Come to the clinic tomorrow so that I can take a look," she responded.

When I got there the doctor looked at me, and I saw her countenance change. She looked concerned. She informed me that because the rash had formed the shape of a butterfly, she wanted me to do a specific test.

"Have you ever done an ANA test?" she politely asked.

I had never heard of an ANA test, let alone had one done.

"What is an ANA test, and am I supposed to have done at some point?" I asked.

She went on to explain that ANA stood for Antinuclear Antibodies and that this test looks for antinuclear antibodies in the blood. She explained that the result will be either positive or negative. If the result was positive, she continued to explain, then it meant that I had an autoimmune disease which means that the antibodies were attacking the healthy cells. If it was negative then we would rule out autoimmune disease and have to do more tests to find the problem.

When I asked why she had asked if I had ever had the ANA test done, she explained that it is recommended for women over 40 years old especially of African and Hispanic descent to do the test, because they are affected in large proportions. That is not to say that women of Asian or Caucasian descent are not affected, or that it does not affect men. I was so confused because none of it made sense.

After the thorough explanation, she asked, *"Can we go ahead and do the test?"*

"Of course," I responded.

She then explained that my insurance was not going to cover the test and that I should pay out of pocket. The test was done and she told me she would call me when the results were ready. I prayed and I waited.

I should point out that by this time there was no doubt in my mind that something was wrong. I looked terrible. My skin was so dry, and the rashes were like nothing I had ever seen in my life. My eyebrows had fallen out and I was unusually tired. The weave that I had on my head was falling off in chunks attached to my hair. That means my hair was falling out from the root as it was still attached to the weave which was very alarming. In a nutshell, I can say, "all hell broke loose". I prayed for the results to be negative, but it looked like the more I prayed, the worse the symptoms became.

"Have you ever prayed, believed, quoted scripture, and instead of things getting better they got worse?"

Earlier I mentioned that none of this made sense to me. This was because, at that time I did not have any health issues and with a background in Foods and Nutrition, I watched what I ate. I was pretty much a very health-conscious person. I exercised regularly, danced a lot, and wore 6-inch high heels with a lot of ease. I traveled a lot around the United States and overseas for business and conferences. I am one of those people described as a "go-getter" and therefore, this baffled both me and my family.

Finally, the doctor called and informed me that the results were ready and I needed to come to the clinic. I asked her if the result was negative or positive, but she said that she would rather not discuss the results over the phone, and gave me an appointment for the next day. The fact that she was not willing to discuss the results over the phone gave me a bad feeling in my stomach. Nevertheless, I kept hoping for the best.

Naturally, I didn't sleep much. The night felt longer than usual. I was tossing and turning, praying under my breath to avoid waking my husband and hoping against hope that the result was negative. Finally, it was morning. I woke up, said my prayers, and got ready to go to the clinic. My husband drove because I wasn't feeling strong enough to drive. On arrival, we were ushered to the doctor's office. The doctor greeted us and asked us to sit. She then turned to me and informed me that the ANA test came back positive. Therefore, I had an autoimmune disease. As to which specific one, that was to be determined by a rheumatologist.

I had more questions than answers. What type of autoimmune disease was this? How did I get it? How will it be cured? It's as though the doctor read my mind. She told me that I needed to undergo more tests to establish what type of autoimmune disease I had because there are several. Those tests needed to be done by a rheumatologist. Therefore, we needed to find one as soon as possible.

Finding a rheumatologist who would see me quickly proved to be a difficult process. Every one of them I called had a long waiting period because of the number of appointments they already had in the books. Days went by, and the longer it took the rashes on my face were increasing, I had lost my eyebrows, and my muscles were weakening so much that I could not open a water bottle. I decided to remove the weave on my hair because my hair was falling out. As I removed the weave, my hair was coming out attached to the weave.

By the time I was done, I was left with a bald head with a few patches of hair in the front part of my head. I called my daughter so that she could see the unbelievable thing that I was experiencing. I then called my husband and he could not believe what he was seeing. At that point, I knew I was in more trouble than I even imagined. These were the signs of trouble. I had to take action immediately, therefore I booked an appointment the very next day to see my primary doctor. She prescribed antibiotics because she was concerned that my skull would get infected.

My hair and skull

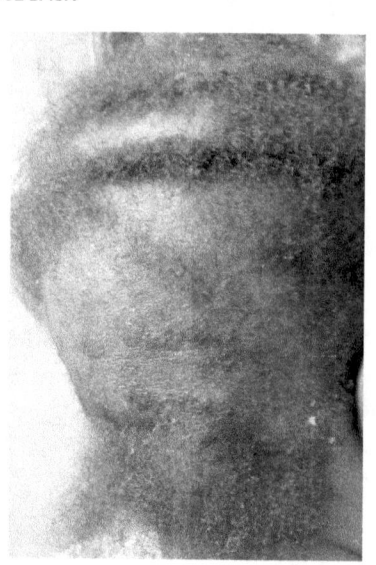

3

The Wait

Getting an appointment with a rheumatologist immediately was a challenge. I soon realized that there are not very many rheumatologists around, and because of that, the wait time was long. Another challenge was finding one who accepted my insurance. Finally, when I found one, the earliest available date was in three months. Clearly, this was not going to work for me because I was in critical condition and the situation was getting worse day by day. I had to make a decision quickly.

While I was looking for a rheumatologist in private practice, I completely forgot that my county hospital had a well-equipped rheumatology department with some of the best rheumatologists in the country. So, after tiring from seeking a rheumatologist in private practice, which felt like looking for a needle in a haystack, I decided to go to my county hospital. I told my husband to drive me straight to the emergency room. Upon arrival, the doctors took one look at me and admitted me immediately. Unbeknown to me, this was the beginning of a long journey.

Upon arrival, the doctors took one look at me and admitted me immediately. Then the research began. This was the beginning of a long journey unbeknown to me.

Before I was wheeled into my room, I closed my eyes and said a prayer, committing my life into the hands of God. I knew one thing for sure; my help would only come from the Lord. I also prayed for the doctors because I knew that the way I was looking, they would definitely need the Lord to give them divine understanding to figure out this "enemy" that had invaded my body. I remember praying Isaiah 54:17, *"no weapon formed against you will prosper, and you will refute every tongue that accuses you. This is the heritage of the servants of the Lord, and this is their vindication from me, declares the Lord."*

Another scripture was, Isaiah 53:5, *"But he was pierced for our transgressions, he was crushed for our iniquities; the punishment that brought us peace was on him and by his wounds, we are healed."*

The doctors knew that I had an autoimmune disease, but they had to figure out which particular autoimmune disease I had. From that point on, I considered whatever it was the enemy of my destiny and I declared an all-out war against it. The journey and fight had just begun.

The day I was admitted, May 2016

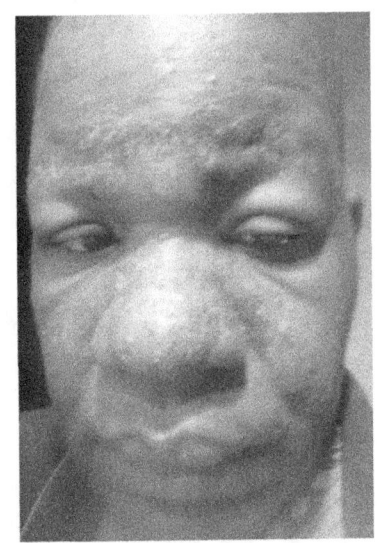

This picture says it all. In a very short period of time, my face had completely been deformed. You could not find any resemblance to any of my photos. I did not know what to make of it. During the taking of this picture, I still had not found a rheumatologist who had time in their schedule to see me. It is frustrating, to say the least when you have everything you need to have, which is insurance, but no doctor to see you. Truly, I am grateful for the county hospital.

4

The Process of Diagnosis

Immediately after being admitted, doctors began the process of diagnosing what was wrong with me. They simply could not go by how I looked physically, even though they had an idea, they had to be sure that there was nothing they were missing. Doctors came in and out of my room running blood work after blood work.

As you see in the picture below, they had to take a biopsy of my skin to confirm they were not missing anything. Specialists of all kinds came in trying to diagnose my condition. I was being treated by the head rheumatologist leading a team of doctors alongside a team of dermatologists. I am so grateful for this.

The state of my skin

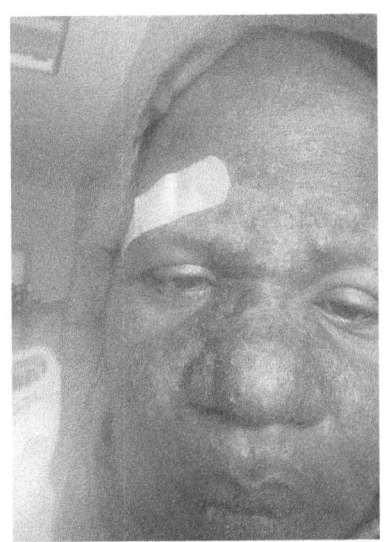

It was about a month from the time the signs showed up to the time I was admitted,. It took the doctors three full days to finally reach the conclusion that I had systemic lupus. That was the first part. The second past was for the rheumatologist and the dermatologist to come together and decide on the medicine that was going to work to control the lupus while clearing my skin.

Having all my doctors under the same roof was a blessing. My medication was a combined effort of both the rheumatologist and the dermatologist. After they decided on the type of medicine and dose of medicines I was to take, I had to stay in the hospital for another three days to make sure I responded well to the medication.

Once the doctors were satisfied and sure that all was well, they discharged me to begin my very long journey to recovery.

5

The Process of Recovery

The process of recovery took a very long and painstaking two and a half years. In those two years, I did not work in my business nor did I take any speaking engagements. I was completely confined to my house. I was required to stay away from the sun because of the medications. The only place I went to was my doctor's appointments with my husband driving me. I completely lost muscle strength. I could not open a water bottle let alone open the car door. It was so devastating because, prior to this I was healthy, walking all the time, eating, and dancing a lot. Now, I could not even take myself to the restroom. My husband had to help me. I am really grateful for my husband.

The side effect of the medication was another challenge I had to deal with. Prior to this, I was one of the people who would not take medicine for my headache. If I had a headache all I did was drink water, rest and make sure that there's enough fresh air flowing in the room. So, you can imagine how difficult it was for me to go from that to taking many bottles of pills. Even my speech and coordination became affected.

Dark Room

My eyes developed a sensitivity to light due to the medication and for that reason, I had to stay in a dark room. Otherwise, my eyes would ache and I would get a migraine. So, for many days, I stayed in my bedroom with the curtains closed. When I used a laptop or a computer, I had to use a screen protector.

My Skin

I was told that the scars on my face would take many years to heal or remain permanent. The scars were really dark as you can see in the pictures below. The dermatologist told me that applying ointment on the skin was not going to clear them because the problem was systemic. Therefore, I had to be patient and wait and see if after a while they would fade.

The dermatologist also told me that moving forward I needed to use sunscreen without fail. I never applied sunscreen because I believed that as a black woman I didn't need to put sunscreen. Still, he made it clear to me that if I didn't put on sunscreen and wear clothes with long sleeves, my skin would be affected because the disease plus the medication made my skin very sensitive to the sun. My life as I knew it had now changed and I was going to have to adjust.

Dancing/Praising as my exercise

In order to gain back muscle strength, the rheumatologist recommended that I exercise. The challenge was, the medication I was taking suppressed my immune system, therefore going to the gym was out of the question. The doctor also warned against carrying weight and strenuous exercises because of muscle weakness. It seemed like the only option I had so it seemed was walking but because I like dancing, I decided to dance every morning to gospel music. This way I was exercising and doing my morning praise.

In the beginning, I was able to dance for only five minutes. Every day I kept adding one more minute. Before long, I was dancing for ten minutes and my muscles were getting stronger. I kept dancing for ten minutes for a while to avoid straining. After about a year, I was able to dance for twenty minutes with no difficulties. This was how I gained back my strength and dancing became my way of exercise to date.

Food

For a long time, I was not able to add weight and the rheumatologist was wondering why I could not add weight. At one point my primary care physician had to get me an appointment with a nutritionist. The nutritionist really helped me understand the measures of different foods that I was supposed to eat and that really helped.

Prayers

Prayer was my anchor. Prayer was my hope. From the very beginning when the rheumatologist told me that there's no cure for systemic lupus, I knew I was going to have to believe God for a miracle, and believing I did. My family and my friends joined me in praying. It wasn't easy because the more we prayed the worse it looked. After 2 years, things started turning for the good. God is faithful.

The Side Effects Affected My ability to Think and Talk at the Same Time

When I started taking the medicine, I was aware of the side effects, and honestly, the side effects were scarier than lupus.

One morning I did something crazy. I took all the medicines and put them on the table and I started praying and speaking to each one of the medicines declaring the side effects null and void.

There comes a time when you have to take drastic measures. One of the side effects was that I no longer had the ability to think and talk simultaneously. I had to think, take time, and then speak. This was rather scary because as a conference speaker, losing my ability to think on my feet was frightening. Thank God that it only lasted a few weeks.

Support System

Those you surround yourself with can break you or make you. They can either help you or frustrate you. I am very blessed to have a group of people around me who are very prayerful and are also very good people.

They did not let me give up and prayed with me. Most of all, they stood with me until a miracle happened. I am grateful for all those who surrounded me and prayed with me relentlessly.

My Family

My husband was great and absolutely amazing throughout this ordeal. When I became completely unable to even use the restroom, he took me to the restroom and helped me shower. He cooked, cleaned, and took me to my appointments for two years and never complained or showed signs of despair. How I thank God for him. When I couldn't pray, he prayed over me and encouraged me. I am forever grateful for my husband.

My children were the reason I was fighting. I wanted to see them graduate and I wanted to see them grow. Our daughter Sifa had not graduated eighth grade and I was determined that I was going to be there for her graduation. Our son was studying in college and I wanted to be there for his graduation. I wanted to see him grow into a man. For this reason, I was fighting and fighting hard and believing in God for a miracle.

Joshua may have been away in college, but Sifa was around to help her dad take care of me. Many times, she stayed with me in the bedroom and brought me anything I needed. When my husband went to work, she was in charge. During the summer, Joshua came home and he was shocked to see how sick I was. I knew the two of them were worried and concerned to say the least so I had to assure them that I was going to be alright.

My brother, Dr.Wycliffe Opii (aka Omosh)

What can I say about my brother? This brother of mine was a source of strength for me. It helped that he is a physician because I needed a doctor that I trusted in my corner. He called every day to encourage me and make sure I took my medicine because he knew I did not like medicine. I would ask him many questions and he patiently answered each one of them. Let me just say, having his voice in my ear helped me fight. I'm forever grateful to God for him.

My Fellowship (The Twelve Springs)

My fellowship went above and beyond. Every month they made sure that fellowship was hosted in our house because I was not in any position to go anywhere. Usually, we met at each other's homes every month, but because of my condition, they chose to host the fellowships at my house, and they did this for over two years. Not only did they bring joy to our home, but they cooked and made sure we were alright. They encouraged my family and did whatever they could to make sure that we felt supported. I must mention their names to make sure it is forever recorded who I am grateful for. Anne Lantey, Paul Lantey, Betty

Ogaye, Liz Oduor, Musi Kiarie, and Eric Kiarie. I am forever grateful.

The Community

For many years, I have lived in Dallas and have had the honor of serving our community in different capacities. I have ministered, MC'd at weddings and dinners, and also spoken in various forums. I not only served my Dallas community, but I have had the privilege and honor to travel the country and serve, especially in women's conferences. When news of my ailment reached the various groups that knew me, they all started interceding for me. Prayers went up from the East Coast to the West Coast, from Up North to the Deep South. I cannot say how grateful I am.

Let me tell you how the news started spreading. When I was admitted to the hospital, one of the nurses came to my room. I will remember her for the rest of my life. After greeting me and making sure that I was settling in, she asked me an interesting question.

"Are you from Kenya?"

"I am," I shrugged, *"why do you ask?"*

"Well, there are times when foreigners or immigrants are admitted in the hospital and they have nobody to take care of them. So, I made it a habit to ask the patient so I can know if there are any relatives they need to call."

I thought that was the kindest gesture ever. She was relieved once I assured her that I had family and that my husband was the one who brought me to the hospital.

She then asked me how long I had lived in Dallas, and I told her and told her that she probably knew me. I was confident of this because of the many events I had served in. I showed her my picture from my phone and she blurted.

"Oh my! You are Evangelist Millicent?" her eyes brimming with sadness.

"Yes," I nodded.

I asked her not to be sad and encouraged her that everything was going to be alright because God is in control. I found the moment to be ironic because now I was the encourager.

She went back to her station and informed another nurse who is also a native of Kenya that she had just seen me and I didn't look good. This second nurse had just seen me the previous weekend and couldn't believe that I was now in the hospital.

When she came to my room, she couldn't help tearing up as she looked at me. She could not believe what she was seeing. I told her there was no need to worry because our God the healer, Jehovah Rapha, is in control.

I asked her to call the first lady of her home church and pleaded that they needed to start praying because I was in the ER and I wasn't looking good. Their first lady then notified some other ladies and the chain began from there. People prayed and prayed and prayed. For this, I am forever grateful. May God bless everyone who prayed.

6

Lessons Learned

Faith is being sure of what you hoped for and certain of the things you do not see. That's what Hebrews 11 tells us, but this scripture is easier said than done. What I mean is that it was easy to believe for my healing when there was hope of getting well.

When the doctor came back with the results after three days of research and told me that what I was suffering from was systemic lupus, I still didn't understand the seriousness of the situation. So, my faith was still intact. My belief for healing was unmoved. After he explained to me exactly what was going on in my body, my mind started racing, but I still was not shaken.

Until he informed me that there was no cure, I felt my legs give way and my faith began to crumble. I needed to encourage myself so I knew one thing for sure—moving forward, I had to control my mind and my tongue. I knew that what I was saying and how I was thinking was going to make the process of my recovery easier or difficult because of the creative ability of those two organs.

I learned that everything from that point depended on me

believing and trusting in the miraculous power of God. I needed a mindset shift. I reminded myself of several scriptures that spoke about healing and immediately started meditating on them.

Always endeavor to feed your mind with the knowledge that you need to succeed. In my case, I am grateful that I had a foundation of the Word of God and understood the Scriptures. This made it possible for me to stand on Scripture and believe when things were hopeless.

Scripture was what I held on to. Galatians 5:22 says, "*the fruits of the Spirit are love, joy, peace, patience, kindness, gentleness, and self-control. Against such things, there is no law.*" This reminded me that I needed to exercise the fruit of patience. It took two years of standing by faith in the promises hidden in the Word of God before I saw significant change.

Proverbs 23:18 says, "*For surely there is an end, and thine expectation shall not be cut off.*"

Believe in God, have faith in the Word of God, and be patient.

Unwavering Faith

By Joshua Nyangon

The first time I saw my mother since she fell ill was when I came back home from college for winter break. On our phone calls her voice was strong, so imagine my surprise when I saw her for the first time.

Her face wore the telltale signs of someone at war, fighting an enemy that was relentless. Holding her frail hands, all I could muster was, *"Why didn't you tell me?"*

We both paused and looked at each other. We both knew why.

My mom has never been one to complain. Her body had betrayed her, but her faith remained un-wavered. My mom never sought sympathy and I knew treating her any different would be an insult.

To many, my mother is many things. However, to me, my mother is everything. She is vigilant and loving. She is an unstoppable force and an unmovable object. She has been and will continue to be my voice of reason and my guiding light.

To my mother, I adore you.

Never Take Life for Granted

By Sifa Nyangon

At the beginning of March 2016, my family and I were doing what we usually do, relaxing, laughing, and enjoying our time together. Then on that same night, my mother's life changed forever. As she began to run her fingers through her beautiful thick hair, I saw the confused look on her face—a palm of her hair in her hands.

She cried out repeatedly, *"No, this can't be my hair falling out."*

A couple of weeks passed, and we noticed a rash growing on my mother's nose that spread out to her cheeks, eyebrows, and forehead forming a butterfly. I was alarmed by what was happening to my mother. At the time, I was in the seventh grade, so imagine a young 14-year old girl handling the stress of her mother's health while also juggling demanding schoolwork. My emotions were an unexplainable rollercoaster. I would go to school happy, then end my day hopeless and crushed by the sorrow of knowing my mother is suffering, and no one can find the cause of her problem.

Over two months, I saw my mother lose her hair, lose muscle strength to a point where she couldn't open a water bottle. She went from 160 to 124 pounds in 42 days and continuously needed assistance walking. She also temporarily lost the ability to drive because it would quickly consume all the energy she had left for the day.

In May 2016, she was admitted to Parkland ER for three days. I was still unsure of what was exactly happening to my mother. I fell into a deep void in my life. My emotions were in despair. Tears were soaking up my pillow as I slept wondering will my mother survive or whether I will I continue living with her. I had to repudiate my emotions from taking over me. My soul was weeping close to falling into depression; however, I kept my faith and stayed strong, believing her health will be restored.

On May 26, 2016, unfortunately, we received the most heart-breaking news when she was unexplainably diagnosed with Systemic Lupus Erythematosus (SLE). The immune system naturally fights off dangerous infections and bacteria to keep the body healthy. An autoimmune disease occurs when the immune system attacks the body because it confuses it for something foreign.

Towards the end of 2016, I witnessed my mother temporarily lose the ability to think and talk at the same time. Speech became an obstacle course. Eye sensitivity weakened over a period of months and lungs and heart at risk.

At the beginning of 2017, treatment began. Treatment consisted of taking several medicines orally and having a portable intravenous therapy pack dangling from her arm, to be pumped with a light yellow liquid medicine substance with a three-inch pointy syringe, every night for six weeks.

Prednisone, one of the several medicines she took, caused a major setback on our journey to good health. Prednisone is a prescription steroid drug. It comes as an immediate-release tablet, a delayed-release tablet, and a liquid solution.

Prednisone weakens your immune system, and a weakened immune system makes you more likely to get infections.

Just when I thought she was getting better, I felt we were walking back to where we started. Prednisone caused a medium, shriveled, puss-drenched boil on her right foot. The infection spread deeper to her foot, going to the bone.

In Mid 2017, she was taken for surgery. Gosh, recovery wasn't the easiest. Can you imagine being immobile for a month with your life pressed on paused, with the anxiousness to press play? Throughout the year, we finally continued to progress.

In 2018, I could feel a new essence in the atmosphere. Almost like I can smell an aroma of a new beginning. Everything my mother lost, she gained back in a better form. Butterfly shaped rashes vanished never to reappear. Hair that was lost grew back curly, baby soft locs. She went from slow brain activity to back to her talkative, intelligent self. Energy and muscle strength were restored like a new pack of batteries. An adult woman weighing the same amount as her 14-year-old daughter gained back her weight to 165 pounds. Gaining back all the abilities she lost, we can say my mother was healed.

Personally, going through a life-threatening situation with my mother took a toll on my life. I've learned to never take anyone's life for granted, to cherish the good moments as much as you can, and to be strong in the weakest point in your life. Yes, my mother is currently in good health, but I desire to hear her say, "I am Lupus free."

www.ingramcontent.com/pod-product-compliance
Lightning Source LLC
Chambersburg PA
CBHW070845220526
45466CB00002B/894